90 All Natural Lung Cancer Meal and Juice Recipes:

These Meals and Juices Will Help You Strengthen Your Immune System to Recover from and Prevent Cancer

By

Joe Correa CSN

COPYRIGHT

© 2017 Live Stronger Faster Inc.

This publication is designed to provide accurate and authoritative information in regard to the subject matter covered. It is sold with the understanding that neither the author nor the publisher is engaged in rendering medical advice. If medical advice or assistance is needed, consult with a doctor. This book is considered a guide and should not be used in any way detrimental to your health. Consult with a physician before starting this nutritional plan to make sure it's right for you.

ACKNOWLEDGEMENTS

This book is dedicated to my friends and family that have had mild or serious illnesses so that you may find a solution and make the necessary changes in your life.

90 All Natural Lung Cancer Meal and Juice Recipes:

These Meals and Juices Will Help You Strengthen Your Immune System to Recover from and Prevent Cancer

By

Joe Correa CSN

CONTENTS

ABOUT THE AUTHOR

After years of Research, I honestly believe in the positive effects that proper nutrition can have over the body and mind. My knowledge and experience has helped me live healthier throughout the years and which I have shared with family and friends. The more you know about eating and drinking healthier, the sooner you will want to change your life and eating habits.

Nutrition is a key part in the process of being healthy and living longer so get started today. The first step is the most important and the most significant.

INTRODUCTION

90 All Natural Lung Cancer Meal and Juice Recipes: These Meals and Juices Will Help You Strengthen Your Immune System to Recover from and Prevent Cancer

By Joe Correa CSN

This book will provide you with valuable juice and meal recipes that will help your body absorb nutrients it needs in order to function properly and fight off all types of diseases including lung cancer. Implementing these recipes into your everyday life will have a powerful effect on your overall health. I honestly believe we have no choice but to forge our own path to wellness through adequate food choices. This primarily refers to fresh fruits and vegetables which are the key to good health. The more we are able to return to eating as nature intended, the better our chances will be of living a cancer-free life.

For lung cancer, your best options are colorful fruits and vegetables. These foods are full of antioxidants, including vitamins A and C which are proven to help fight off this type of cancer. Fruits like berries and vegetables like tomatoes, winter squash, and bell peppers are particularly good and your juices and meals should be based on them. These foods, when combined correctly, can have powerful effects.

These lung cancer preventing juice and meal recipes are great tasting and healthy. Prevent and heal lung cancer using these wonderful recipes.

90 ALL NATURAL LUNG CANCER MEAL AND JUICE RECIPES: THESE MEALS AND JUICES WILL HELP YOU STRENGTHEN YOUR IMMUNE SYSTEM TO RECOVER FROM AND PREVENT CANCER

JUICES

1.   **Avocado Beet Juice**

Ingredients:

1 cup of avocado, chopped

1 cup of beets, trimmed

1 large carrot, sliced

1 small ginger knob

¼ tsp turmeric, ground

2 oz water

Preparation:

Peel the avocado and cut lengthwise in half. Remove the pit and cut into bite-sized pieces. Fill the measuring cup and reserve the rest in the refrigerator.

Trim off the green parts of the beets. Slightly peel and cut into thin slices. Fill the measuring cup and refrigerate the rest.

Wash and peel the carrot. Cut into bite-sized pieces and set aside.

Peel the ginger knob and cut into small pieces. Set aside.

Now, combine avocado, beets, carrot, and ginger in a juicer. Process until well juiced and transfer to a serving glass. Stir in the turmeric and water and refrigerate for 15 minutes before serving.

Enjoy!

Nutrition information per serving: Kcal: 265, Protein: 5.9g, Carbs: 33.4g, Fats: 21.8g

2.   Pomegranate Cantaloupe Juice

Ingredients:

1 cup of pomegranate seeds

1 large wedge of cantaloupe

1 small green apple, cored

1 small ginger knob, sliced

1 oz of water

Preparation:

Cut the top of the pomegranate fruit using a sharp paring knife. Slice down to each of the white membranes inside of the fruit. Pop the seeds into a measuring cup and set aside.

Cut the cantaloupe in half. Scrape out the seeds and cut one one large wedge. Peel and chop into small pieces. Wrap the rest in a plastic foil and refrigerate for later.

Wash the apple and cut lengthwise in half. Remove the core and cut into bite-sized pieces. Set aside.

Peel the ginger and cut into small pieces. Set aside.

Now, combine pomegranate, cantaloupe, apple, and ginger in a juicer. Process until well juiced and transfer to a serving glass. Add some water to adjust the bitterness, if needed.

Refrigerate for 10-15 minutes before serving.

Nutrition information per serving: Kcal: 162, Protein: 3.1g, Carbs: 45.3g, Fats: 1.5g

3. Grapefruit Apricot Juice

Ingredients:

2 whole grapefruits

1 cup of collard greens, chopped

2 whole apricots, pitted

¼ tsp of turmeric, ground

Preparation:

Peel the grapefruits and divide into wedges. Cut each wedge in half and set aside.

Wash the collard greens thoroughly under cold running water. Drain and chop into small pieces. Set aside.

Wash the apricots and cut lengthwise in half. Remove the pit and cut into bite-sized pieces. Set aside.

Now, combine grapefruit, collard greens, and apricots in a juicer and process until juiced. Transfer to a serving glass and stir in the turmeric.

Refrigerate for 10 minutes before serving.

Enjoy!

Nutrition information per serving: Kcal: 208, Protein: 5.8g, Carbs: 62.1g, Fats: 1.2g

4. Honeydew Melon Cucumber Juice

Ingredients:

1 large wedge of honeydew melon

1 cup of cucumber, sliced

1 cup of whole cranberries

2 large strawberries

1 oz coconut water

Preparation:

Cut melon lengthwise in half. Scoop out the seeds and then wash the melon. Cut one wedge and peel it. Cut into bite-sized pieces and set aside.

Wash the cucumber and cut into thin slices. Fill the measuring cup and reserve the rest for later. Set aside.

Using a small colander, rinse well the cranberries. Drain and set aside.

Wash the strawberries and remove the stems. Chop into small pieces and set aside.

Now, combine melon, cucumber, cranberries, and strawberries in a juicer. Process until well juiced. Transfer to a serving glass and add few ice cubes.

Serve immediately.

Nutrition information per serving: Kcal: 96, Protein: 1.8g, Carbs: 31.4g, Fats: 0.6g

5.   Cauliflower Artichoke Juice

Ingredients:

1 cup of cauliflower, chopped

1 medium artichoke, chopped

1 whole lemon, peeled and halved

1 small zucchini, thinly sliced

1 small ginger knob, chopped

¼ tsp salt

Preparation:

Trim off the outer layer of the cauliflower. Cut into bite-sized pieces and wash it. Fill the measuring cup and sprinkle with some salt. Set aside.

Trim off the outer layers of the artichoke using a sharp paring knife. Cut into bite-sized pieces and set aside.

Peel the lemon and cut lengthwise in half. Set aside.

Wash the zucchini and thinly slice it. Set aside.

Peel the ginger knob and chop into small pieces. Set aside.

Now, combine cauliflower, artichoke, lemon, zucchini, and ginger in a juicer. Process until well juiced.

Transfer to a serving glass and refrigerate for 15 minutes before serving.

Enjoy!

Nutrition information per serving: Kcal: 82, Protein: 8.4g, Carbs: 28.9g, Fats: 1.1g

6.   Pineapple Banana Juice

Ingredients:

1 cup of pineapple chunks

1 large banana, sliced

1 cup of blackberries

1 whole lime, peeled

1 oz of water

Preparation:

Using a sharp paring knife, cut the top of the pineapple. Gently remove all hard skin and slice it into thin slices. Fill the measuring cup and reserve the rest for later.

Peel the banana and cut into thin slices. Set aside.

Place the blackberries in a small colander and wash under cold running water. Slightly drain and set aside.

Peel the lime and cut lengthwise in half. Set aside.

Now, combine pineapple, banana, blackberries, and lime in a juicer. Process until well juiced. Transfer to a serving glass and add some ice before serving.

Enjoy!

Nutrition information per serving: Kcal: 222, Protein: 4.5g, Carbs: 70.2g, Fats: 1.4g

7. Bell Pepper Tomato Juice

Ingredients:

1 large red bell pepper, chopped

1 medium whole tomato, chopped

1 cup of watercress, torn

1 rosemary sprig

1 oz of water

Preparation:

Wash the bell pepper and cut lengthwise in half. Remove the seeds and chop into small pieces. Set aside.

Wash the tomato and place in a small bowl. Chop into small pieces and make sure to reserve the tomato juice while cutting. Set aside.

Wash the watercress thoroughly under cold running water. Slightly drain and torn with hands into small pieces. Set aside.

Now, combine bell pepper, tomato, and watercress in a juicer and process until juiced. Transfer to a serving glass and stir in the water and reserved tomato juice. Sprinkle with rosemary and serve immediately.

Enjoy!

Nutrition information per serving: Kcal: 56, Protein: 3.5g, Carbs: 15.1g, Fats: 0.7g

8.   Pumpkin Carrot Juice

Ingredients:

1 cup of pumpkin, cubed

1 large carrot, sliced

1 cup of cucumber, sliced

1 large orange, peeled and wedged

1 small ginger knob, chopped

Preparation:

Cut the top of a pumpkin. Cut lengthwise in half and then scrape out the seeds. Cut one large wedge and peel it. Cut into small cubes and fill the measuring cup. Reserve the rest in the refrigerator.

Wash and peel the carrot. Cut into thin slices and set aside.

Wash the cucumber and cut into thin slices. Fill the measuring cup and reserve the rest for later. Set aside.

Peel the orange and divide into wedges. Cut each wedge in half and set aside.

Peel the ginger knob and cut into small pieces. Set aside.

Now, combine pumpkin, carrot, cucumber, orange, and ginger in a juicer. Process until well juiced. Transfer to a serving glass and add some ice.

Serve immediately.

Nutrition information per serving: Kcal: 130, Protein: 4.1g, Carbs: 39.1g, Fats: 0.6g

9.   Spinach Radish Juice

Ingredients:

1 cup of fresh spinach, torn

2 large radishes, chopped

1 cup of cucumber, sliced

1 cup of arugula, torn

¼ tsp turmeric, ground

Preparation:

Wash the spinach thoroughly under cold running water. Slightly drain and torn with hands. Set aside.

Wash the radishes and trim off the green parts. Peel and cut into thin slices. Set aside.

Wash the cucumber and cut into thin slices. Set aside.

Wash the arugula and torn with hands. Set aside.

Now, combine spinach, radish, cucumber, and arugula in a juicer and process until juiced. Transfer to a serving glass and stir in the turmeric.

Refrigerate for 15 minutes before serving.

Nutrition information per serving: Kcal: 53, Protein: 9.4g, Carbs: 15.3g, Fats: 1.1g

10.   Apple Plum Juice

Ingredients:

1 medium-sized Red Delicious apple, cored

1 whole plum, cored

1 large banana, peeled and chunked

¼ tsp of cinnamon, ground

2 oz of water

Preparation:

Wash the apple and cut lengthwise in half. Remove the core and cut into bite-sized pieces. Set aside.

Wash the plum and cut in half. Remove the pit and cut into bite-sized pieces. Set aside.

Peel the banana and cut into small chunks. Set aside.

Now, combine apple, plum, and banana in a juicer and process until well juiced. Transfer to a serving glass and stir in the water and cinnamon.

Add few ice cubes before serving and enjoy!

Nutrition information per serving: Kcal: 238, Protein: 2.5g, Carbs: 68.4g, Fats: 1.1g

11.   Broccoli Beet Juice

Ingredients:

2 cups of broccoli, chopped

1 cup of beets, trimmed and chopped

1 cup of fresh parsley, torn

1 cup of celery, chopped

¼ tsp of turmeric, ground

¼ tsp ginger, ground

Preparation:

Wash the broccoli and trim off the outer layers. Chop into small pieces and set aside.

Wash and peel the beets. Trim off the green ends and chop into bite-sized pieces. Fill the measuring cup and reserve the rest for later.

Rinse the parsley under cold running water and slightly drain. Torn with hands into small pieces and set aside.

Wash the celery stalks and chop it into bite-sized pieces. Fill the measuring cup and set aside.

Now, combine broccoli, beets, parsley, and celery in a juicer and process until juiced. Transfer to a serving glass and stir in the turmeric and ginger.

Refrigerate for 10 minutes before serving.

Nutrition information per serving: Kcal: 109, Protein: 9.8g, Carbs: 31.8g, Fats: 1.5g

12.   Watermelon Peach Juice

Ingredients:

1 cup of watermelon, cubed

1 large peach, pitted and chopped

1 medium-sized green apple, cored and chopped

1 small banana, chunked

¼ tsp of cinnamon, ground

Preparation:

Cut the watermelon in half. Cut one large wedge and wrap the rest in a plastic foil and refrigerate. Peel the slice and cut into small cubes. Remove the pits and fill the measuring cup. Set aside.

Wash the peach and cut lengthwise in half. Remove the pit and chop into bite-sized pieces. Set aside.

Peel the banana and cut into small chunks. Set aside.

Now, combine watermelon, peach, apple, and banana in a juicer and process until juiced. Transfer to a serving glass and stir in the cinnamon.

Add some ice and serve immediately!

Nutrition information per serving: Kcal: 260, Protein: 4.4g, Carbs: 73.9g, Fats: 1.3g

13.   Yellow Pepper Zucchini Juice

Ingredients:

1 large yellow bell pepper, chopped

1 medium-sized zucchini, sliced

1 cup of fresh basil, chopped

1 large carrot, sliced

¼ tsp of ginger, ground

Preparation:

Wash the bell pepper and cut lengthwise in half. Remove the stem and seeds. Cut into small pieces and set aside.

Wash the zucchini and cut into small chunks. Set aside.

Wash the basil thoroughly under cold running water. Slightly drain and chop into small pieces. Set aside.

Wash and peel the carrot. Cut into thin slices and set aside.

Now, combine pepper, zucchini, basil, and carrot in a juicer and process until juiced. Transfer to a serving glass and stir in the ginger. Add some water if needed.

Refrigerate for 10 minutes before serving.

Nutrition information per serving: Kcal: 94, Protein: 5.6g, Carbs: 25.4g, Fats: 1.3g

14.   Strawberry Spinach Juice

Ingredients:

1 cup of strawberries, chopped

1 cup of spinach, torn

1 whole lemon, peeled

1 whole lime, peeled

1 tbsp honey, raw

2 oz of water

Preparation:

Wash the strawberries and remove the stems. Cut into bite-sized pieces and set aside.

Wash the spinach thoroughly under cold running water. Slightly drain and torn into small pieces. Set aside.

Peel the lemon and lime. Cut each fruit lengthwise in half and set aside.

Now, combine strawberries, spinach, lemon, and lime in a juicer and process until juiced. Transfer to a serving glass and stir in the water and honey.

Garnish with some mint, but it's optional.

Refrigerate for 15 minutes before serving.

Enjoy!

Nutrition information per serving: Kcal: 81, Protein: 5.8g, Carbs: 27.8g, Fats: 1.4g

15.   Asparagus Cauliflower Juice

Ingredients:

1 cup of asparagus, chopped

1 cup of cauliflower, chopped

1 cup of celery, chopped

1 cup of cucumber, sliced

¼ tsp of turmeric, ground

¼ tsp of cayenne pepper, ground

Preparation:

Wash the asparagus under cold running water. Trim off the woody ends and chop into bite-sized pieces. Set aside.

Wash the cauliflower and trim off the outer leaves. Chop into small pieces and fill the measuring cup. Reserve the rest for later.

Wash the celery and chop into bite-sized pieces. Set aside.

Wash the cucumber and cut into thin slices. Fill the measuring cup and reserve the rest in the refrigerator.

Now, combine asparagus, cauliflower, celery, and cucumber in a juicer and process until juiced. Transfer to a serving glass and stir in the turmeric and cayenne pepper.

Serve immediately.

Nutrition information per serving: Kcal: 52, Protein: 6.1g, Carbs: 15.4g, Fats: 0.7g

16.   Cherry Lemon Juice

Ingredients:

1 cup of fresh cherries, pitted

1 whole lemon, peeled

1 medium-sized artichoke, chopped

1 medium-sized apple, cored

¼ tsp of cinnamon, ground

Preparation:

Wash the cherries using a large colander. Cut each in half and remove the pits. Set aside.

Peel the lemon and cut lengthwise in half. Set aside.

Wash the artichoke and trim off the outer, hard leaves. Cut into bite-sized pieces and set aside.

Wash the apple and cut lengthwise in half. Remove the core and cut into bite-sized pieces. Set aside.

Now, combine cherries, lemon, artichoke, and apple in a juicer and process until juiced. Transfer to a serving glass and stir in the cinnamon.

Refrigerate for 10 minutes before serving.

Nutrition information per serving: Kcal: 205, Protein: 7.2g, Carbs: 66.2g, Fats: 0.9g

17.   Mango Blackberry Juice

Ingredients:

1 cup of mango, chunked

1 cup of blackberries

1 large banana, chunked

1 large orange, peeled

¼ tsp of cinnamon, ground

Preparation:

Wash the mango and cut into small chunks. Fill the measuring cup and reserve the rest for later.

Place the blackberries in a colander and wash under cold running water. Slightly drain and set aside.

Peel the banana and cut into small chunks. Set aside.

Peel the orange and divide into wedges. Cut each wedge in half and set aside.

Now, combine mango, blackberries, banana, and orange in a juicer and process until juiced. Transfer to a serving glass and stir in the cinnamon.

Add few ice cubes and serve immediately.

Nutrition information per serving: Kcal: 296, Protein: 6.6g, Carbs: 91.2g, Fats: 2.1g

18.   Avocado Carrot Juice

Ingredients:

1 cup of avocado, chunked

1 large carrot, chopped

1 cup of collard greens, torn

1 cup of Romaine lettuce, shredded

1 whole cucumber, sliced

¼ tsp of ginger, ground

Preparation:

Peel the avocado and cut lengthwise in half. Remove the pit and cut into small chunks. Fill the measuring cup and reserve the rest in the refrigerator.

Wash and peel the carrot. Cut into thin slices and set aside.

Combine collard greens and lettuce in a large colander. Wash thoroughly under cold running water. Drain and shred. Set aside.

Wash the cucumber and cut into thin slices. Fill the measuring cup and reserve the rest for later. Set aside.

Now, combine avocado, carrot, collard greens, lettuce, and cucumber in a juicer and process until juiced. Transfer to a serving glass and stir in the ginger.

Refrigerate for 10 minutes before serving.

Nutrition information per serving: Kcal: 271, Protein: 7.3g, Carbs: 34.1g, Fats: 22.8g

19.　Raspberry Pear Juice

Ingredients:

1 cup of raspberries

1 large pear, cored

1 whole plum, pitted and chopped

1 medium-sized Granny Smith's apple, cored

¼ tsp of cinnamon, ground

1 oz of coconut water

Preparation:

Wash the raspberries using a small colander. Slightly drain and set aside.

Wash the pear and cut lengthwise in half. Remove the core and cut into small pieces. Set aside.

Wash the plum and cut in half. Remove the pit and set aside.

Wash the apple and cut in half. Remove the core and cut into bite-sized pieces. Set aside.

Now, combine raspberries, pear, plum, and apple in a juicer and process until well juiced. Transfer to a serving glass and stir in the cinnamon and coconut water. Add some crushed ice and serve immediately.

Enjoy!

Nutrition information per serving: Kcal: 239, Protein: 3.5g, Carbs: 79.9g, Fats: 1.6g

20.   Guava Mango Juice

Ingredients:

1 whole guava, chopped

1 cup of mango, chunked

1 tbsp of liquid honey

1 whole lime, peeled

1 cup of cucumber, sliced

1 medium-sized Golden Delicious apple, cored

Preparation:

Peel the guava using a sharp paring knife. Cut into bite-sized pieces and set aside.

Wash and peel the mango. Cut into small chunks and set aside.

Peel the lime and cut lengthwise in half. Set aside.

Wash the cucumber and cut into thin slices. fill the measuring cup and reserve the rest in the refrigerator.

Wash the apple and cut lengthwise in half. Remove the core and cut into bite-sized pieces. Set aside.

Now, combine guava, mango, lime, cucumber, and apple in a juicer and process until well juiced. Transfer to a serving glass and stir in the honey. Add some crushed ice and serve immediately.

Nutrition information per serving: Kcal: 211, Protein: 3.7g, Carbs: 61.1g, Fats: 1.5g

21.   Blueberry Spinach Juice

Ingredients:

1 cup of blueberries

1 cup of fresh spinach, chopped

1 whole lime, peeled

1 medium-sized orange

1 oz coconut water

Preparation:

Place the blueberries in a colander and wash under cold running water. Slightly drain and set aside.

Wash the spinach thoroughly and drain. Chop into small pieces and set aside.

Peel the lime and cut lengthwise in half. Set aside.

Peel the orange and divide into wedges. Cut each wedge in half and set aside.

Now, combine blueberries, spinach, lime, and orange in a juicer and process until well juiced. Transfer to a serving glass and stir in the coconut water.

Sprinkle with some fresh mint. However, it's optional.

Enjoy!

Nutrition information per serving: Kcal: 158, Protein: 8.5g, Carbs: 48.1g, Fats: 1.5g

22.   Pepper Broccoli Juice

Ingredients:

1 large green bell pepper, chopped

1 cup of broccoli, chopped

1 cup of Brussels sprouts, halved

1 whole lime, peeled

2 large carrots, sliced

¼ tsp turmeric, ground

Preparation:

Wash the bell pepper and cut lengthwise in half. Remove the stem and seeds. Chop into small pieces and set aside.

Wash the broccoli and Brussels sprouts. Trim off the wilted and outer leaves. Place in a heavy-bottomed pot and add water enough to cover all. Bring it to a boil and then remove from the heat. Drain well and chop into small pieces. Set aside to cool completely.

Peel the lime and cut lengthwise in half. Set aside.

Wash and peel the carrots. Cut into thin slices and set aside.

Now, combine bell pepper, broccoli, Brussels sprouts, lime, and carrots in a juicer and process until juiced. Transfer to a serving glasses and stir in the turmeric. Add some water, if needed.

Sprinkle with some salt, but it's optional.

Nutrition information per serving: Kcal: 122, Protein: 8.5g, Carbs: 39.1g, Fats: 1.2g

23.   Cantaloupe Grapefruit Juice

Ingredients:

1 cup of cantaloupe, cubed

1 whole grapefruit

1 cup of fresh mint, torn

¼ tsp of cinnamon, ground

1 oz coconut water

Preparation:

Cut the cantaloupe in half. Scoop out the seeds and flesh. Cut and peel one large wedge. Chop into chunks and fill the measuring cup. Reserve the rest of the cantaloupe in a refrigerator.

Peel the grapefruit and divide into wedges. Cut each wedge in half and set aside.

Wash the mint thoroughly and torn with hands into small pieces. Set aside.

Now, combine cantaloupe, grapefruit, and mint in a juicer. Process until well juiced.

Transfer to a serving glass and stir in the cinnamon and coconut water. Add some ice and serve immediately.

Nutrition information per serving: Kcal: 144, Protein: 4.2g, Carbs: 42.6g, Fats: 0.9g

24. Pomegranate Apple Juice

Ingredients:

1 cup of pomegranate seeds

1 medium-sized Granny Smith's apple, cored

1 large banana, chunked

1 tbsp of liquid honey

1 oz of water

Preparation:

Cut the top of the pomegranate fruit using a sharp paring knife. Slice down to each of the white membranes inside of the fruit. Pop the seeds into a measuring cup and set aside.

Wash the apple and cut lengthwise in half. Remove the core and cut into bite-sized pieces. Set aside.

Peel the banana and cut into small chunks. Set aside.

Now, combine pomegranate, apple, and banana in a juicer and process until juiced. Transfer to a serving glass and stir in the honey and water.

Serve cold.

Nutrition information per serving: Kcal: 243, Protein: 3.6g, Carbs: 70.1g, Fats: 1.8g

25.   Zucchini Basil Juice

Ingredients:

1 medium-sized zucchini, chopped

1 cup of fresh basil, torn

1 cup of cucumber, sliced

1 cup of red leaf lettuce, torn

1 cup of avocado, cut into bite-sized pieces

Preparation:

Peel the zucchini and chop into small pieces. Set aside.

Combine basil and lettuce in a large colander and rinse under cold running water. Drain and torn with hands into small pieces. Set aside.

Peel the avocado and cut lengthwise in half. Remove the pit and cut into bite-sized pieces. Fill the measuring cup and reserve the rest in the refrigerator.

Wash the cucumber and cut into thin slices. Fill the measuring cup and refrigerate for later.

Now, combine zucchini, basil, lettuce, avocado, and cucumber in a juicer. Process until well juiced. Transfer to a serving glass and add some ice.

Serve immediately.

Nutrition information per serving: Kcal: 234, Protein: 6.7g, Carbs: 21.7g, Fats: 22.3g

26.   Banana Peach Juice

Ingredients:

1 cup of banana, sliced

1 large peach, pitted and chopped

1 small green apple, cored and chopped

¼ tsp of cinnamon, ground

1 oz of coconut water

1 tbsp of mint, finely chopped

Preparation:

Peel the bananas and cut into thin slices. Fill the measuring cup and reserve the rest in the refrigerator.

Wash the peach and cut lengthwise in half. Remove the pit and cut into bite-sized pieces. Set side.

Wash the apple and cut in half. Remove the core and chop into small pieces. Set aside.

Now, combine bananas, peach, and apple in a juicer and process until well juiced. Transfer to a serving glass and stir in the cinnamon and coconut water. Add some crushed ice and sprinkle with finely chopped mint for some extra taste.

Enjoy!

Nutrition information per serving: Kcal: 362, Protein: 5.5g, Carbs: 104g, Fats: 1.7g

27.   Swiss Chard-Tomato Juice

Ingredients:

1 cup of cherry tomatoes, halved

1 cup of Swiss chard, torn

1 cup of basil, torn

1 cup of beets, trimmed

¼ tsp of balsamic vinegar

¼ tsp of salt

1 oz of water

Preparation:

Wash the cherry tomatoes and remove the green stems. Cut in half and fill the measuring cup. Reserve the rest in the refrigerator for some other juice.

Combine Swiss chard and basil in a large colander and rinse thoroughly under cold running water. Drain and torn with hands into small pieces. Set aside.

Wash the beets and trim off the green parts. Cut into thin slices and fill the measuring cup. Reserve the rest for later.

Now, combine cherry tomatoes, Swiss chard, basil, and beets in a juicer and process until juiced. Transfer to a serving glass and stir in the vinegar, salt, and water.

Serve immediately.

Nutrition information per serving: Kcal: 72, Protein: 5.1g, Carbs: 21.6g, Fats: 0.7g

28. Pear Apricot Juice

Ingredients:

1 large pear, chopped

3 whole apricots, pitted

1 cup of pomegranate seeds

1 medium-sized orange, wedged

¼ tsp of cinnamon, ground

Preparation:

Wash the pear and cut lengthwise in half. Cut into bite-sized pieces and set aside.

Wash the apricots and cut each in half. Remove the pit and cut into small pieces. Set aside.

Cut the top of the pomegranate fruit using a sharp paring knife. Slice down to each of the white membranes inside of the fruit. Pop the seeds into a measuring cup and set aside.

Peel the orange and divide into wedges. Cut each wedge in half and set aside.

Now, combine pear, apricots, pomegranate seeds, and orange in a juicer. Process until well juiced. Transfer to a serving glass and stir in the cinnamon.

Refrigerate for 10 minutes before serving.

Nutrition information per serving: Kcal: 253, Protein: 4.9g, Carbs: 78.3g, Fats: 1.9g

29.   Kale Zucchini Juice

Ingredients:

1 cup of fresh kale, chopped

1 medium-sized zucchini, chopped

1 whole lemon, peeled

1 whole lime, peeled

1 cup of fresh mint, torn

Preparation:

Rinse the kale thoroughly under cold running water. Drain and chop into small pieces. Set aside.

Wash the zucchini and cut into small pieces. Set aside.

Peel the lemon and lime. Cut lengthwise in half and set aside.

Wash the mint and chop into small pieces. Set aside.

Now, combine kale, zucchini, lemon, lime, and mint in a juicer. Process until well juiced. Transfer to a serving glass and add some crushed ice.

Serve immediately.

Nutrition information per serving: Kcal: 79, Protein: 7g, Carbs: 24.7g, Fats: 1.7g

30.   Kiwi Apricot Juice

Ingredients:

2 whole kiwis, peeled and halved

3 whole apricots, chopped

1 large green apple, cored

1 large banana, chunked

Preparation:

Peel the kiwi and cut lengthwise in half. Set aside.

Wash the apricots and cut in half. Remove the pits and cut into small pieces. Set aside.

Wash the apple and cut lengthwise in half. Remove the core and cut into bite-sized pieces. Set aside.

Peel the banana and cut into small chunks. Set aside.

Now, combine kiwi, apricots, apple, and banana in a juicer and process until juiced. Transfer to a serving glass and add some ice.

Serve immediately.

Nutrition information per serving: Kcal: 313, Protein: 5.4g, Carbs: 91g, Fats: 1.9g

31.   Mango Mint Juice

Ingredients:

1 cup of mango, chunked

1 cup of fresh mint, torn

1 small Red Delicious apple, cored

1 medium-sized peach, pitted

Preparation:

Peel the mango and cut into small chunks. Fill the measuring cup and reserve the rest in the refrigerator.

Wash the mint thoroughly under cold running water and torn with hands. Set aside. You can soak mint in hot water for 2 minutes, but it's optional.

Wash the apple and cut lengthwise in half. Remove the core and cut into bite-sized pieces. Set aside.

Wash the peach and cut in half. Remove the pit and cut into small pieces. Set aside.

Now, combine mango, mint, apple, and peach in a juicer and process until well juiced. Transfer to a serving glass and add few ice cubes.

Serve immediately.

Nutrition information per serving: Kcal: 227, Protein: 4.1g, Carbs: 64.9g, Fats: 1.6g

32.   Orange Fennel Juice

Ingredients:

1 medium-sized orange, peeled

1 medium-sized pear, chopped

1 cup of fennel, chopped

1 whole lemon, peeled

¼ tsp of cinnamon, ground

1 oz of coconut water

Preparation:

Peel the orange and divide into wedges. Cut each wedge in half and set aside.

Wash the pear and cut in half. Remove the core and cut into small pieces. Set aside.

Trim off the outer wilted layers of the fennel. Roughly chop it and fill the measuring cup. Reserve the rest for later.

Peel the lemon and cut lengthwise in half. Set aside.

Now, combine orange, pear, fennel, and lemon in a juicer and process until well juiced. Transfer to a serving glass and stir in the cinnamon and coconut water.

Refrigerate for 15 minutes before serving.

Enjoy!

Nutrition information per serving: Kcal: 156, Protein: 3.6g, Carbs: 54.2g, Fats: 0.7g

33.   Beet Raspberry Juice

Ingredients:

1 cup of beets, sliced

1 cup of raspberries

1 whole lemon, peeled

1 medium-sized pear, chopped

1 oz of water

Preparation:

Wash the beets and trim off the green parts. Cut into thin slices and fill the measuring cup. Reserve the rest for later.

Rinse well the raspberries using a small colander. Drain and set aside.

Peel the lemon and cut lengthwise in half. Set aside.

Wash the pear and cut in half. Remove the core and cut into bite-sized pieces. Set aside.

Now, combine beets, raspberries, lemon, and pear in a juicer and process until juiced. Transfer to a serving glass and stir in the water.

Refrigerate for 10 minutes before serving.

Nutrition information per serving: Kcal: 165, Protein: 4.9g, Carbs: 60.2g, Fats: 1.4g

34.   Sweet Potato Celery Juice

Ingredients:

1 cup of sweet potatoes, cubed

1 cup of celery, chopped

1 medium-sized apple, cored

1 medium-sized orange, peeled

1 tbsp of fresh mint, torn

Preparation:

Peel the sweet potato and cut into small cubes. Fill the measuring cup and reserve the rest for later. Set aside.

Wash the celery and cut into bite-sized pieces. Set aside.

Wash the apple and cut lengthwise in half. Remove the core and cut into bite-sized pieces. Set aside.

Peel the orange and divide into wedges. Cut each wedge in half and set aside.

Now, combine sweet potatoes, celery, apple, and orange in a juicer. Process until well juiced. Transfer to a serving glass and sprinkle with mint.

Add some crushed ice and serve immediately.

Nutrition information per serving: Kcal: 236, Protein: 4.7g, Carbs: 67.8g, Fats: 0.7g

35.   Tomato Spinach Juice

Ingredients:

1 medium whole tomato, chopped

1 cup of fresh spinach, torn

1 medium-sized carrot, sliced

1 cup of celery, chopped

¼ tsp of salt

¼ tsp of balsamic vinegar

Preparation:

Wash the tomato and place in a small bowl. Cut into bite-sized pieces. Make sure to reserve the tomato juice while cutting. Set aside.

Wash the spinach thoroughly under cold running water. Torn into small pieces and set aside.

Wash and peel the carrot. Cut into thin slices and set aside.

Wash the celery and chop into small pieces. Set aside.

Now, combine tomato, spinach, carrot, and celery in a juicer and process until juiced. Transfer to a serving glass and stir in the salt, vinegar, and reserved tomato juice.

Serve cold.

Nutrition information per serving: Kcal: 72, Protein: 8.4g, Carbs: 21.2g, Fats: 1.4g

36. Strawberry Lime Juice

Ingredients:

1 cup of strawberries, chopped

1 whole lime, peeled

1 small Granny Smith's apple, cored

1 whole lemon, peeled

2 oz coconut water

¼ tsp cinnamon, ground

Preparation:

Wash the strawberries and remove the stems. Cut into bite-sized pieces and fill the measuring cup. Reserve the rest for later.

Peel the lime and lemon. Cut each fruit in half and set aside.

Wash the apple and cut lengthwise in half. Remove the core and cut into small pieces. Set aside.

Now, combine strawberries, lime, lemon, and apple in a juicer and process until juiced. Transfer to a serving glass and stir in the coconut water and cinnamon.

Add some crushed ice and serve immediately.

Nutrition information per serving: Kcal: 122, Protein: 2.4g, Carbs: 39.7g, Fats: 0.9g

37.   Pineapple Orange Juice

Ingredients:

1 cup of pineapple, chunked

1 large orange, peeled

½ cup of spinach, torn

3 Brussels sprouts, halved

Preparation:

Using a sharp paring knife, cut the top of the pineapple. Gently remove all hard skin and slice it into thin slices. Fill the measuring cup and reserve the rest for later.

Peel the orange and divide into wedges. Cut each wedge in half and set aside.

Wash the spinach thoroughly under cold running water and torn with hands. Set aside.

Wash the Brussels sprouts and trim off the wilted leaves. Cut each in half and set aside.

Now, combine pineapple, orange, spinach, and Brussels sprouts in a juicer and process until well juiced. Transfer to a serving glass and refrigerate for 15 minutes before serving.

Enjoy!

Nutrition information per serving: Kcal: 172, Protein: 7.9g, Carbs: 52.7g, Fats: 1.1g

38. Carrot Celery Juice

Ingredients:

1 large carrot, sliced

1 cup of celery, chopped

1 whole lemon, peeled

1 small Golden Delicious apple, cored

¼ tsp turmeric, ground

¼ tsp ginger, ground

Preparation:

Wash and peel the carrot. Cut into small slices and set aside.

Wash the celery and cut into small pieces. Set aside.

Peel the lemon and cut lengthwise in half. Set aside.

Wash the apple and cut in half. Remove the core and cut into bite-sized pieces. Set aside.

Now, combine carrot, celery, lemon, and apple in a juicer and process until juiced. Transfer to a serving glass and stir in the water, turmeric, and ginger. If you like, add some crushed ice.

Serve immediately.

Nutrition information per serving: Kcal: 105, Protein: 2.4g, Carbs: 32.8g, Fats: 0.7g

39.   Pear Cabbage Juice

Ingredients:

1 large pear, chopped

1 cup of purple cabbage, chopped

1 whole lemon, peeled

1 whole cucumber, sliced

Preparation:

Wash the pear and cut lengthwise in half. Remove the core and chop into small pieces. Set aside.

Wash the cabbage thoroughly under cold running water. Drain and chop into small pieces. Set aside.

Peel the lemon and cut lengthwise in half. Set aside.

Wash the cucumber and cut into thin slices. Set aside.

Now, combine pear, cabbage, lemon, and cucumber in a juicer. Process until well juiced. Transfer to a serving glass and serve immediately.

Enjoy!

Nutrition information per serving: Kcal: 173, Protein: 4.7g, Carbs: 57.9g, Fats: 0.9g

40. Cauliflower Tomato Juice

Ingredients:

1 cup of cauliflower, chopped

1 medium-sized tomato, chopped

½ cup of spring onions, chopped

½ cup of basil, torn

1 cup of cucumber, sliced

1 oz of water

Preparation:

Trim off the outer leaves of the cauliflower. Wash it and cut into small pieces. Fill the measuring cup and reserve the rest for later. Set aside.

Wash the tomato and place in a small bowl. Chop into small pieces and reserve the tomato juice while cutting. Set aside.

Wash the spring onions and basil. Chop into small pieces. Set aside.

Wash the cucumber and cut into thin slices. Fill the measuring cup and reserve the rest for later. Set aside.

Now, combine cauliflower, tomato, spring onions, basil, and cucumber in a juicer and process until well juiced. Transfer to a serving glass and stir in the water.

Serve cold.

Nutrition information per serving: Kcal: 51, Protein: 4.4g, Carbs: 13.9g, Fats: 0.7g

41.   Cantaloupe Strawberry Juice

Ingredients:

1 cup of cantaloupe, chopped

1 cup of strawberries, chopped

1 cup of banana, chunked

2 whole plums, chopped

¼ tsp of cinnamon, ground

Preparation:

Cut the cantaloupe in half. Scrape out the seeds and cut one one large wedge. Peel and chop into small pieces and fill the measuring cup. Wrap the rest in a plastic foil and refrigerate for later.

Wash the strawberries and remove the stems. Cut into bite-sized pieces and set aside.

Peel the banana and cut into chunks. Fill the measuring cup and reserve the rest. Set aside.

Wash the plums and cut each in half. Remove the pits and cut into small pieces. Set aside.

Now, combine cantaloupe, strawberries, banana, and plums in a juicer and process until juiced. Transfer to a serving glass and stir in the cinnamon.

Add some crushed ice and serve immediately.

Nutrition information per serving: Kcal: 249, Protein: 4.8g, Carbs: 73.1g, Fats: 1.5g

42.   Swiss Chard Kale Juice

Ingredients:

2 cups of Swiss chard, torn

1 cup of fresh kale, torn

1 cup of pomegranate seeds

1 large orange, peeled

1 small Granny Smith's apple, cored

Preparation:

Combine Swiss chard and kale in a large colander. Rinse under cold running water and drain. Torn into small pieces and set aside.

Cut the top of the pomegranate fruit using a sharp paring knife. Slice down to each of the white membranes inside of the fruit. Pop the seeds into a measuring cup and set aside.

Peel the orange and divide into wedges. Cut each wedge in half and set aside.

Wash the apple and cut lengthwise in half. Remove the core and cut into bite-sized pieces. Set aside.

Now, combine Swiss chard, kale, pomegranate seeds, orange, and apple in a juicer and process until juiced. Transfer to a serving glass and add few ice cubes.

Serve immediately.

Nutrition information per serving: Kcal: 227, Protein: 7.9g, Carbs: 66.1g, Fats: 2.3g

43.   Pineapple Mango Juice

Ingredients:

1 cup of pineapple, chunked

1 cup of mango, chopped

1 cup of kale, torn

1 large orange, peeled

1 small ginger knob, chopped

Preparation:

Using a sharp paring knife, cut the top of the pineapple. Gently remove all hard skin and cut it into small chunks. Fill the measuring cup and reserve the rest for later.

Peel the mango and chop into small pieces. Fill the measuring cup and reserve the rest for later. Set aside.

Wash the kale thoroughly under cold running water. Drain and torn into small pieces. Set aside.

Peel the orange and divide into wedges. Cut each wedge in half and set aside.

Peel the ginger knob and cut into small pieces. Set aside.

Now, combine pineapple, mango, kale, orange, and ginger in a juicer and process until juiced. Transfer to a serving glass and refrigerate for 15 minutes before serving.

Enjoy!

Nutrition information per serving: Kcal: 258, Protein: 6.9g, Carbs: 74.9g, Fats: 1.7g

44.   Pepper Cabbage Juice

Ingredients:

1 large red bell pepper, chopped

1 cup of purple cabbage, chopped

1 cup of beets, sliced

1 cup of fresh spinach, torn

3 cherry tomatoes, halved

¼ tsp of salt

Preparation:

Wash the bell pepper and cut lengthwise in half. Remove the stem and seeds. Cut into small pieces and set aside.

Combine cabbage and spinach in a large colander. Rinse thoroughly under cold running water and drain. Torn into small pieces and set aside.

Wash the beets and trim off the green parts. Peel and cut into thin slices and fill the measuring cup. Reserve the rest for later.

Wash the cherry tomatoes and remove the stems. Cut into halves and set aside.

Now, combine bell pepper, cabbage, beets, spinach, and tomatoes in a juicer and process until juiced. Transfer to a serving glass and stir in the salt.

Serve immediately.

Nutrition information per serving: Kcal: 134, Protein: 11.5g, Carbs: 39.1g, Fats: 1.8g

45.   Blueberry Cucumber Juice

Ingredients:

1 cup of blueberries

1 cup of cucumber, sliced

1 cup of strawberries, chopped

1 cup of fresh mint, torn

1 large carrot, sliced

¼ tsp of cinnamon, ground

Preparation:

Wash the blueberries using a small colander. Drain and set aside.

Wash the cucumber and cut into thin slices. Fill the measuring cup and reserve the rest in the refrigerator.

Wash the strawberries and remove the stems. Chop into small pieces and set aside.

Wash the mint thoroughly under cold running water. Drain and torn into small pieces. Set aside.

Wash and peel the carrot. Cut into thin slices and set aside.

Now, combine blueberries, cucumber, strawberries, mint, and carrot in a juicer. Process until well juiced.

Transfer to a serving glass and stir in the cinnamon. Add some crushed ice and serve immediately!

Nutrition information per serving: Kcal: 141, Protein: 4g, Carbs: 45g, Fats: 1.3g

46.   Grape Cherry Juice

Ingredients:

2 cups of green grapes

1 cup of frozen cherries, thawed

1 small banana, peeled

1 whole lime, peeled

1 tbsp of coconut water

Preparation:

Rinse the grapes under cold running water and remove the stems. Set aside.

Peel the banana and cut into chunks. Set aside.

Peel the lime and cut lengthwise in half. Set aside

Now, combine grapes, cherries, banana, and lime in a juicer and process until juiced. Transfer to a serving glass and stir in the coconut water.

Serve immediately.

Nutrition information per serving: Kcal: 292, Protein: 4.1g, Carbs: 82.9g, Fats: 1.3g

47.   Lemon Leek Juice

Ingredients:

1 whole lemon, peeled

1 whole leek, chopped

1 whole lime, peeled

1 large orange, peeled

1 small green apple, cored

Preparation:

Peel the lemon and lime. Cut each fruit lengthwise in half and set aside.

Wash the leek and chop into small pieces. Set aside.

Peel the orange and divide into wedges. Cut each wedge in half and set aside.

Wash the apple and cut in half. Remove the core and cut into small pieces. Set aside.

Now, combine lemon, leek, lime, orange, and apple in a juicer and process until juiced. Transfer to a serving glass and refrigerate for 15 minutes before serving.

Enjoy!

Nutrition information per serving: Kcal: 205, Protein: 4.5g, Carbs: 62.9g, Fats: 0.9g

48.   Avocado Radish Juice

Ingredients:

1 cup of avocado, cubed

3 large radishes, chopped

1 small zucchini, sliced

1 cup of celery, chopped

1 cup of cucumber, sliced

¼ tsp of salt

1 oz of water

Preparation:

Peel the avocado and cut in half. Remove the pit and cut into small cubes. Fill the measuring cup and reserve the rest for later.

Wash the radishes and cut into small pieces. Set aside.

Wash the zucchini and cut into thin slices. Set aside.

Wash the celery and chop it into bite-sized pieces. Set aside.

Wash the cucumber and cut into thin slices. Fill the measuring cup and reserve the rest for later. Set aside.

Now, combine avocado, radishes, zucchini, celery, and cucumber in a juicer and process until juiced. Transfer to a serving glass and stir in the salt and water.

Serve cold.

Nutrition information per serving: Kcal: 235, Protein: 5.6g, Carbs: 22.3g, Fats: 22.6g

49.   Mango Kiwi Juice

Ingredients:

1 cup of mango, chopped

1 whole kiwi, peeled

1 small Grany Smith's apple, cored

1 small ginger knob, peeled

2 oz of coconut water

Preparation:

Peel the mango and cut into small pieces. Fill the measuring cup and reserve the rest for later.

Peel the kiwi and cut lengthwise in half. Set aside.

Wash the apple and cut lengthwise in half. Remove the core and cut into small pieces. Set aside.

Peel the ginger knob and cut into small pieces. Set aside.

Now, combine mango, kiwi, apple, and ginger in a juicer and process until juiced. Transfer to a serving glass and stir in the coconut water. Add some crushed ice and serve immediately.

Enjoy!

Nutrition information per serving: Kcal: 196, Protein: 2.8g, Carbs: 55.5g, Fats: 1.3g

50.   Broccoli Pumpkin Juice

Ingredients:

1 cup of broccoli, chopped

1 cup of pumpkin, cubed

1 whole lemon, peeled

1 cup of fennel, chopped

1 cup of cucumber, sliced

Preparation:

Wash the broccoli and trim off the outer leaves. Cut into bite-sized pieces and fill the measuring cup. Reserve the rest for later.

Cut the top of a pumpkin. Cut lengthwise in half and then scrape out the seeds. Cut one large wedge and peel it. Cut into small cubes and fill the measuring cup. Reserve the rest in the refrigerator.

Peel the lemon and cut lengthwise in half. Set aside.

Trim off the outer wilted layers of the fennel. Roughly chop it and fill the measuring cup. Reserve the rest for later.

Wash the cucumber and cut into thin slices. Fill the measuring cup and reserve the rest in the refrigerator. Set aside.

Now, combine broccoli, pumpkin, lemon, fennel, and cucumber in a juicer and process until well juiced. Transfer to a serving glass and add some crushed ice.

Serve immediately.

Nutrition information per serving: Kcal: 196, Protein: 2.8g, Carbs: 55.5g, Fats: 1.3g

MEALS

1.   Super Green Eggs

Ingredients:

6 eggs

½ cup milk

¼ cup sour cream

¼ cup extra virgin olive oil

1 small onion

¼ cup cheese of choice

1 16 oz. bag collard greens

¼ teaspoons red pepper flakes

Pinch of salt

How to Prepare:

Beat the eggs, salt and pepper, milk and sour cream in a bow. Sauté thinly chopped onions in a skillet with one tablespoon of olive oil. Add the egg mixture and let cook slowly until the eggs are almost firm. Add the collard greens, cheese, and the pepper flakes. Fold the eggs over the collard greens and cook until the greens are soft and the eggs are firm.

2.   Painted Beans and Greens

Ingredients:

1 can precooked pinto beans

1 16 oz. bag of collard greens

1 cup chicken stock

Pinch salt and pepper

1 tbsp. red pepper flakes

1 tbsp. olive oil

1 clove garlic

1 tsp. chili powder

How to Prepare:

Boil a pot of salted water and add the collard greens, boil till soft. Drain. In a skillet sauté garlic and oil. Add onions and cook until mixture is clear.

Add the chicken stock and add the pinto beans that have been rinsed and drained. Heat thoroughly and add the drained collard greens. Add the chili powder, salt pepper, and pepper flakes. Cook until the collards are soft.

This dish is also good served the next day after the flavors have blended.

3.   Collard Green Salad

Ingredients:

1 16 oz. bag collard greens

1 bag mixed salad vegetables

1 tomato diced

1 red pepper diced

1 cucumber

1 red onion

3 tbsp. Herb flavored Olive oil (olive oil infused with rosemary and basil especially)

2 tbsp. Red Wine vinegar

Salt and Pepper to taste.

How to Prepare:

Combine all ingredients in a large bowl and mix.

Eat chilled.

4.   Green Toast

Ingredients:

1 Loaf Italian Bread

1 tbsp. olive oil

1 clove garlic

1 tsp. parsley

1 tsp. basil

1 tsp. oregano

Pinch of salt and pepper

1 bag collard greens cooked and drained

1 lb. shredded mozzarella cheese

How to Prepare:

Slice Bread lengthwise. Using a pestle mash the spices and garlic with the olive oil until paste is formed. Spread the paste on the bread.

Strain the collard greens in your hands and dry with a towel. Remove as much moisture as possible. Layer the collard greens over the paste.

Add the mozzarella on top and broil until the cheese melts. Eat warm

5.   Green Pasta

Ingredients:

3 eggs

3 cups flour

1 cup water

1 tsp. salt

8 oz. collard greens cooked and drained.

How to Prepare:

Drain the collard greens after boiling until all the water is out of them.

In a mixer add eggs, water and salt. Slowly add the flour while mixing constantly on a low speed. When the dough comes together it is time to add the collard greens. Incorporate them thoroughly into the dough.

Let the dough sit for about 20 minutes covered with a damp cloth.

Using a pasta machine work the dough through the machine until the desired shape appears. Dry until ready to cook.

6.   Green Pasta with Lemon Pepper Sauce

Ingredients:

Green Pasta

3 Lemons (One sliced into thin slices, two juiced)

1 tsp. black pepper

1 garlic glove

2 tsp. olive oil

¼ cup parmesan Cheese, Grated

How to Prepare:

Cook pasta in a large pot with salted water. Dry pasta should take about 6 minutes for an 'al dente' texture.

To prepare the sauce, sauté the garlic in the olive oil. Slowly add the juice of 2 lemons and the slices of one lemon. Add the salt and black pepper. Add 1 tablespoon of the grated cheese.

Add the al dente pasta to the skillet and add some the pasta water to combine as a sauce.

Add more parmesan cheese to your preference.

7.   Green Soup

Ingredients:

1-quart chicken stock

1 16 oz. bag collard greens

1 cup cubed bread pieces

1 12 oz. bag of shredded carrots

1 small onion, minced

1 tbsp. minced garlic

1 tbsp. olive oil

¼ cup mushrooms, washed, sliced

How to Prepare:

Boil and drain collard green in a pan of salted water. Drain.

In a soup pan, add olive oil and sauté minced garlic, minced onion, and sliced mushrooms. Add the carrots and collard greens.

Add the stock to the pan and heat through. Add the cubed bread and serve.

8.   Green Grilled Chicken Breast

Ingredients:

4 skinless chicken breasts

8 oz. collard greens boiled and drained

1 garlic clove, minced

1 tbsp. olive oil

2 slices mozzarella cheese

2 slices roasted red peppers

1 tsp. crushed red pepper flakes

Salt and paper to taste

How to Prepare:

Grill chicken breast until just about cooked. Remove from grill.

In a sauté pan add the minced garlic in the olive oil and add the drained collard greens. Add the pepper flakes. Remove from pan.

Transfer the chicken to the skillet and add the salt and pepper. Layer the collard greens, roasted red peppers and top with cheese. Cook until the cheese is melted and the wellness is to your liking.

9.   Green Rice

Ingredients:

2 cups cooked wild rice

1 16 oz. bag of collard greens cooked and chopped

1-cup chicken stock

3 slices turkey bacon, chopped

1 can black beans, precooked

1 small onion chopped

1 glove garlic chopped

1 tbsp. olive oil

Salt and pepper to taste

How to Prepare:

Sauté turkey bacon, olive oil, garlic and onion. Add chicken stock. Season with salt and pepper and transfer to a large pan. To this large pan, add the precooked beans and cooked wild rice. Heat for 5 minutes, while stirring well. Add salt and pepper to taste, then serve.

10.   Red and Green Salad

Ingredients:

1 bunch Broccoli stem cut off

1-cup cherry tomatoes

2 cups cooked tortellini

1 small can sliced back olives

1 small red onion

1 tbsp. olive oil

1 tsp. red wine vinegar

1 tsp. oregano

Pinch of salt and pepper

How to Prepare:

Blanch broccoli crowns, cut cherry tomatoes in half, drain olives, and chop the red onion.

Add the cooked tortellini and all ingredients in a large bowl. Toss with oil, vinegar and oregano. Add salt and pepper to taste. Chill before serving.

11.   Broccoli Soup

Ingredients:

1 cup chicken stock

1 bunch broccoli stems removed

1 glove garlic, minced

1-cup heavy cream

½ cup cheddar cheese

1 small onion chopped

Pinch of salt and pepper

How to Prepare:

In a soup pan, sauté onion and garlic. Add the broccoli florets and continue to cook until the broccoli is soft. Add salt and pepper.

Add the chicken stock and boil at low heat. Add heavy cream and slowly warm the soup to high heat for 4 minutes. Add the cheddar cheese and slowly bring back to a low heat. Allow to cool, then serve at desired temperature.

12.   Chicken, Rice and Broccoli

Ingredients:

2 cups cooked wild rice

2 chicken breast cubed

1 tbsp. Olive oil

1 Garlic clove, minced

1 broccoli crown

1 lemon, sliced

Pinch of salt and pepper

How to Prepare:

Clean broccoli crown and chop until the pieces are uniform. In a steamer add the broccoli and sliced lemon into the water. Steam for five minutes or until the desired level of softness of the broccoli.

Saute the olive oil with garlic in a pan and add the chicken cubes. Add the pinch of salt and pepper to taste. Cook for about 10 minutes until chicken shows no sign of pink and is completely white in the center of the cubes.

Add the broccoli crowns and toss with the chicken cubes.

In large bowl, pour over the wild rice, then serve.

13.   Chicken and Broccoli

Ingredients:

4 chicken thighs

1 broccoli crown cut into florets

2 large russet potatoes, washed.

Salt and paper to taste

6 chipotle onions, minced

1 tsp. olive oil

How to Prepare:

Sauté the thighs to crisp the crust. Add to the baking pan with potatoes sliced into ¼ inch slices, and minced chipotle onions. Add salt and Pepper to taste. Add olive oil and the remaining oil from the sauté pan.

After 30 minutes in a 350 degree F oven, add the broccoli and toss to blend. Finish cooking until the chicken is cooked completely and the potatoes are soft, then serve.

14.   Broccoli Cheese cakes

Ingredients:

1 crown of broccoli

½ cup grated Parmesan cheese

2 eggs

1 tsp. salt

1 cup flavored breadcrumbs

1 tbsp. olive oil

How to Prepare:

Steam broccoli florets in a water and lemon steamer. Allow to cool, then pulse in a mixer until the consistency of large breadcrumbs. Add eggs, cheese, salt and pulse again. When mixed add the breadcrumbs.

Heat the olive oil in a skillet. With an ice cream scooper, scoop out a portion of the broccoli/breadcrumb mix and flatten on the skillet. Fry until crispy on the one side and then flip. Fry on the other side until crispy. Serve with your favorite dipping sauce.

15.   Broccoli Chicken Farfalle

Ingredients:

1 lb. farfalle pasta

1 broccoli floret

2 cups cooked chicken, squared

2 garlic cloves, crushed

2 tbsp. red pepper flakes

2 tbsp. olive oil

Salt and pepper to taste

Grated Cheese

How to Prepare:

While the salted pasta water is boiling, sauté the crushed garlic clove in olive oil in a frying pan. Add the broccoli floret and the squared, cooked chicken to the sauté and cook for 2 minutes, then set aside.

Cook the farfalle pasta until desired texture, then drain. Then combine the pasta, broccoli, and chicken together and mix. Top with the grated cheese and red pepper flakes, then serve.

16.   Broccoli Muffins

Ingredients:

1 broccoli crown chopped fine

1 onion chopped fine

½ cup chopped carrots

6 eggs

½ cup cheddar cheese, shredded

2 cups flour

2 tsp. baking powder

1 tbsp. sugar

1 tsp. salt

How to Prepare:

In a large bowl beat the eggs. Add the vegetables and mix thoroughly. Add the shredded cheddar cheese, flour, baking powder, sugar and salt, and mix well.

Scoop into muffin cup baking tins.

Bake at 350 degrees F for 30 minutes.

Allow to cool and then serve.

17.   Roasted Broccoli

Ingredients:

1 crown broccoli cut into florets

1 lemon, juiced

Pinch of salt and pepper

Pinch garlic powder

½ tsp. Chili powder

1-tbsp. olive oil

How to Prepare:

Preheat oven to 400 degrees. In a large bowl, toss broccoli florets with olive oil, garlic powder, salt, pepper and chili powder.

Place tossed broccoli florets on a baking pan and roast for 5 minutes. Then turn and finish roasting for another 3 minutes.

Remove from the oven, and allow to cool. Toss with the lemon juice, then serve.

18.   Honey Orange Chicken

Ingredients:

2 chicken breast, cubed and dusted with flour

1 orange, juiced

1 tbsp. olive oil

½ cup honey

1 tbsp. sesame seeds

2 cups cooked rice of your choice

Pinch of salt and pepper

How to Prepare::

Sauté chicken cubes in olive oil to get a dark brown coating on the cubes. Transfer to a baking pan.

In a small bowl, mix the orange juice and honey. Add sesame seeds, then drizzle over chicken cubes.

Bake covered for 20 minutes at 350 degrees F or until the cubes are white and done in the center. Add salt and pepper to taste.

Serve over cooked rice of your choice.

19.   Buffalo Style Cod Fish

Ingredients:

4 cod filets coated with cornmeal

¼ cup hot sauce

¼ cup warmed olive oil

Pinch of salt and pepper to taste

How to Prepare:

Warm the olive oil and hot sauce together in a saucepan.

Dip the coated cod filets in the mixture and place on a baking sheet.

Brush remaining mixture to fully coat the filets.

Bake covered for 10 minutes at 350 degrees F. Serve with sides of choice, such as celery and carrot sticks with bleu cheese dressing.

20.   Squash and Beet salad

Ingredients:

1-cup butternut squash roasted

1-cup beets roasted

1 green apple, chopped

½ cup pecans

2 cups arugula

1 cup orange sections

1 orange, juiced

How to Prepare:

Toss the arugula, green apple, squash, beets and pecans in a bowl. Add the orange sections. Dress with the orange juice. Chill to allow the flavors to infuse each other.

21.   Orange Sections salad

Ingredients:

1 cup orange sections

1 sliced red onion

2 cups salad greens of choice

½ cup shredded carrots

1 cup sliced tomatoes

1 tbsp. olive oil

½ tbsp. balsamic vinegar

Salt and pepper to taste

How to Prepare:

In a large salad bowl, mix the salad greens, orange sections, onion slices, shredded carrots, and sliced tomatoes. Let them rest for a few minutes. In a small bowl, mix the olive oil and balsamic vinegar together, then toss over the salad, and serve cold preferably.

22. Orange Rice

Ingredients:

2 cups rice cooked of your choice

1 small onion chopped

1 small pepper chopped

1-cup broccoli in small pieces

½ cup shredded carrots

1 orange, juiced

½ tbsp. olive oil

Pinch of salt and pepper

How to Prepare:

Heat olive oil in a saucepan and add onions. Cook till onions are clear. Add broccoli, pepper, carrots and cook until tender. Add orange juice and heat for 1 minute. Add salt and pepper. Add rice to the saucepan and stir till well blended. Keep covered and cook on low heat for 5 minutes.

Serve warm. You may add a protein such as cooked chicken or cod, as your prefer.

23.   Chicken a la orange

Ingredients:

1 roasting chicken with the inners removed and washed.

1 whole garlic glove

4 oranges, juiced

1 spring rosemary

3 basil leaves

1 tbsp. olive oil

Pinch of salt and pepper

How to Prepare:

In a crock-pot place half of the orange juice. Place the whole garlic glove, spring rosemary, and basil leaves in the cavity of the chicken. Place the chicken in the crock pot and add the salt and pepper. Pour the olive oil. Pinch small holes in the chicken and pour the other half of the orange juice over the top of the chicken. Let cook for six hours, then serve.

24.   Citrus Lobster Salad

Ingredients:

1 cup of lobster meat. This can be frozen or removed from a fresh steamed lobster

1-cup orange slices

1 small red onion chopped

½ cup shredded carrots

1-cup arugula

2 tbsp. lemon juice

1 tsp. horseradish

2 tbsp. olive oil

How to Prepare:

In a large salad bowl, mix the arugula, orange slices, shredded carrots, and chopped onions. Add lobster meat on top of salad mixture.

Dress the salad lightly with olive oil, lemon juice and dot with horseradish, then serve.

25.　Eggs and Avocado and Tuna

Ingredients:

3 hard-boiled eggs

1 avocado

Pinch of salt and pepper

1 can tuna in oil

How to Prepare:

Clean boiled eggs and chop. Clean out avocado and cut into bite size pieces. In a medium bowl, mix the chopped eggs with the avocado and add the tuna with the oil from the can. Mix lightly, adding the salt and pepper, then serve.

26.   French Toast Bake

Ingredients:

8 eggs

½ cup milk

1 loaf of bread of your choice

1 tbsp. olive oil

½ cup maple syrup

1 tsp. vanilla extract

How to Prepare:

The night before soak the loaf of bread in milk and let it rest in the refrigerator overnight. When ready to prepare, place the soaked bread on a baking pan. In a medium bowl, beat the eggs with ½ cup of milk, add the vanilla extract and olive oil, and pour on top of loaf of bread to cover completely.

Bake at 350 degrees F for 10 minutes then remove from oven. Serve warm with maple syrup.

27. Egg Bake

Ingredients:

8 eggs

1-cup milk

1 pinch salt and pepper

1 package hash browns

1 package turkey sausage, precooked

1 small green pepper, chopped

½ cup cheddar cheese, shredded

How to Prepare:

In a baking pan, layer the sausage on the bottom, then layer the hash browns on top of the sausage.

In a medium bowl, beat the eggs, add milk, salt and pepper, peppers, and the shredded cheddar cheese. Pour onto the pan over the potatoes and allow seeping in between the potatoes. Bake for 10 minutes

This can be left overnight in the refrigerator and baked the next day or it can be baked at this point.

28.   Italian Cod

Ingredients:

4 cod filets

2 boiled russet potatoes, peeled

1-cup green beans steamed

1 small red onion chopped

1 small red pepper chopped

1 clove garlic chopped

Pinch of salt and pepper

2 tbsp. olive oil

1 tbsp. red wine vinegar

How to Prepare:

Sauté the codfish in a frying pan with olive oil until it flakes apart. Slice the codfish filets into small flakes.

Dice the peeled, boiled potatoes into medium size cubes. Steam green beans to the crispness that you prefer, then allow to cool. In a large bowl, mix the green beans, potato cubes, onions, chopped peppers and chopped garlic.

Add the cod filets flakes and toss with olive oil and vinegar. Serve warm or cold.

29. Egg Soup

Ingredients:

2 cups chicken stock

2 eggs

½ cup Parmesan cheese

½ cup shredded carrots

¼ tsp. garlic powder

¼ tsp. salt and pepper

How to Prepare:

Heat chicken stock with shredded carrots until it boils. Add salt and pepper.

In a small bowl, beat the eggs and add to the boiling chicken stock while stirring. Boil for 2 minutes, then add Parmesan cheese. Remove from heat and serve at desired temperature.

30.　Egg Salad Stuffed Tomatoes

Ingredients:

6 hard-boiled eggs, chopped

1 avocado chopped in small pieces

½ cup sour cream

1 chopped onion

½ cup chopped celery

½ cup chopped carrots

1 lime, juiced

4 medium size tomatoes cored

How to Prepare:

In a medium bowl mix the chopped eggs with the chopped onion, carrots and celery. Then add the avocado pieces and pour the lime juice into the bowl. Dress with sour cream, then stuff each of the tomatoes with the filling and enjoy. May add salt and pepper to your taste.

31.   Frittatas

Ingredients:

8 eggs

½ cup milk

1 small onion chopped

1-cup mozzarella cheese, grated

½ cup mushrooms sliced

½ cup red pepper strips

1 baked potato

2 tbsp. olive oil

¼ cup parmesan cheese

How to Prepare:

In a large mixing bowl whisk the eggs, add a dash of salt and pepper and Parmesan cheese.

In a large saucepan with olive oil, add the onions and sauté. Add the mushrooms, red pepper strips and sauté till slightly tender. Add a pinch of salt and pepper to your taste. Pour the egg mixture to the saucepan and gently stir. Top with grated mozzarella cheese. Bake at 350 degrees F for 5 minutes then serve and enjoy.

32.   The Best French toast

Ingredients:

1 loaf of bread

4 eggs

½ cup milk

Dash of salt and pepper

½ tsp. vanilla extract

2 tbsp. olive oil

½ tsp. cinnamon

¼ cup maple syrup

How to Prepare:

Pour the olive oil on a large frying pan and place on medium heat. Whisk the eggs, milk, salt and vanilla together in a medium bowl with a flat bottom. Slice the loaf of bread into ½ inch thick slices. Dip each slice into the egg mixture on the flat bottom allowing it to rest in the mixture on both sides for 2 seconds. Then place each dipped bread slice on the large frying pan and cook until they are light brown on both sides and set aside. Serve with maple syrup or cinnamon and enjoy.

33.   Cod Fish Special

Ingredients:

1 lb. of codfish filets

1 tbsp. olive oil

1 lemon, sliced

½ cup of capers

1 sliced onion

1 small can of black olives sliced

1 small tomato sliced

Flour to coat the filets

How to Prepare:

Line a large baking dish with the cod filets that have been coated with flour. Place the sliced onion, black olives, tomato slices, capers on top and around the cod filets and then drizzle everything with the olive oil.

Cover with aluminum foil and bake for 10 minutes at 350 degrees F. Remove foil and bake for another 2 minutes. Serve warm with lemon on the side.

34.   Stuffed Cod

Ingredients:

6 cod filets

1 cup cooked spinach

1 cup bread crumbs seasoned

½ cup Parmesan cheese

1 egg

1 lemon, sliced

1 tbsp. olive oil

How to Prepare:

In a medium bowl, mix the cooked spinach with the seasoned bread cubes, egg, and parmesan cheese until uniform and firm texture is reached. Spoon out a tablespoon of the spinach mixture and place on the center of each fillet. Carefully wrap the filet around the mixture. Place in a large oven pan and drizzle with olive oil and hint of salt and pepper. Bake for 15 minutes at 350 degrees F. Cod should flake when touched with a fork. Serve with lemon on the side and enjoy.

35.   Orange Cod

Ingredients:

4 cod filets

1 sliced blood orange

½ tsp. garlic powder

1 tbsp. olive oil

Hint of salt and pepper

1 lemon, sliced

How to Prepare:

Arrange the cod filets on an 8 x 12 baking dish. Add a hint of salt and pepper and garlic powder. Sprinkle with olive oil and bake for 8 minutes at 350 degrees F. Remove from oven and top with the slices of blood orange. Complete cooking for 2 additional minutes until cod flakes when touched with a fork. Serve with lemon on the side and enjoy.

36.   Baked Cod Fish

Ingredients:

4 cod filets

1 tbsp. olive oil

1 small tomato, sliced

1 small lemon, sliced

1 tsp. chili powder

Hint of salt and Pepper

How to Prepare:

Layer filets in a baking dish and cover with slices of tomatoes, onion, and lemon.

Drizzle with olive oil and salt, pepper and chili powder. Bake uncovered for 10 minutes at 350 degrees F.

37.   Tuna Melt

Ingredients:

1 can of tuna, in oil

4 slices mozzarella cheese

1 sliced tomato

4 Croissants

1 tsp. olive oil

How to Prepare:

Heat the olive oil on a skillet on low heat. Slice the croissants and place the bottom slice on the pan with the tender area facing up. Spread each of the 4 croissant bottom slices on the tender side with a slice of mozzarella cheese, a slice of tomato, and tuna. Then drizzle some olive oil on top. Cover each bottom slice with the top slice of the croissant and flip holding both side of the sandwich. Cook until the cheese melts and enjoy.

38.   Turkey pepperoni Egg Scramble

Ingredients:

4 eggs slightly beaten

¼ cup milk

6 slices turkey pepperoni, precooked

1 small pepper diced

1 small onion chopped into small pieces

1 tbsp. olive oil

Salt and pepper

How to Prepare:

In a small bowl, beat the eggs. Then heat the olive oil on a medium-sized frying pan at low heat. Sauté the onions, peppers, and turkey pepperoni slices until tender. Add the eggs and the milk, and mix in the pan until uniform. Cook until egg scramble is tender to your taste.

39.   Cod Potato Salad

Ingredients:

4 cod filets cubed

2 baked potatoes, cubed

1 small onion sliced

1 cup mixed sweet peppers sliced

1 tbsp. olive oil

1 cup celery, washed and chopped

Pinch of salt and pepper

How to Prepare:

Sauté onion and peppers in olive oil until the onions are clear. Add salt and pepper. Mix well. Add cod cubes and cook until the cod flakes at the touch of a fork.

In a large salad bowl, combine the baked potato cubes, chopped celery with the cooked cod cubes, and serve hot or cold as per your preference.

40.   Egg Battered Cod

Ingredients:

2 eggs

¼ cup cornmeal

1 tsp. Italian Seasoning

4 cod filets

1 tbsp. olive oil

1 lemon, wedges

How to Prepare:

In a medium bowl, beat the eggs and add cornmeal and Italian seasonings. Mix well. Mixture will be thick but liquid.

Coat the cod filets with the egg mixture.

Heat the olive oil in a large frying pan and add the coated cod filets. Cook on medium heat until the egg mixture on the cod filets turns a light brown. Serve with lemon wedges and enjoy

ADDITIONAL TITLES FROM THIS AUTHOR

70 Effective Meal Recipes to Prevent and Solve Being Overweight: Burn Fat Fast by Using Proper Dieting and Smart Nutrition

By

Joe Correa CSN

48 Acne Solving Meal Recipes: The Fast and Natural Path to Fixing Your Acne Problems in Less Than 10 Days!

By

Joe Correa CSN

41 Alzheimer's Preventing Meal Recipes: Reduce or Eliminate Your Alzheimer's Condition in 30 Days or Less!

By

Joe Correa CSN

70 Effective Breast Cancer Meal Recipes: Prevent and Fight Breast Cancer with Smart Nutrition and Powerful Foods

By

Joe Correa CSN

www.ingramcontent.com/pod-product-compliance
Lightning Source LLC
Chambersburg PA
CBHW030251030426
42336CB00009B/340